Jecca's

STORY

THE FOUNDING OF
CAMPDEN HOME NURSING

Jecca Brook
1937 – 2020

Published by David Brook, Chipping Campden

Design by Loose Chippings
Pan's Place, Chipping Campden, Gloucestershire, GL55 6AU
www.loosechippings.org

Hardback ISBN 978-1-907991-16-5

Contents

Foreword

by David Brook, Jecca's Husband

In February 1990 Jecca (Jessica) and I moved to Chipping Campden in the Cotswolds. With her wide range of nursing experience she already had the idea of setting up a local scheme for nursing the terminally ill in their own homes and in her "Story" she describes the start and development of Campden Home Nursing from 1990 until her retirement in 2004. The scheme is financed by fund-raising in the community and receives no money from the government.

Complementing hospices for care of the dying, home nursing provides care where and when it is sorely needed and saves the NHS and hospices beds and finance.

For Jecca to have set up Campden Home Nursing and provided an example for three further schemes in this area is truly remarkable and an outstanding life-time achievement.

David Brook
March 2021

Introduction

by Jecca Brook

I knew from the age of seven that I wanted to be a nurse, and this book is about where my vocation led me.

Having already cared for my mother at home during her last year of life, in 1989 I travelled to Ottawa to nurse my dying father through his final six weeks of life. I was able to keep him in his own home because I was a trained palliative care nurse.

During the long flight home afterwards, sleep was elusive, and I was pondering on the experience of making my parents' end of life as comfortable, homely and personal as possible, and how such care might be extended to others in my community. I duly discussed my idea with my family, who supported it with great enthusiasm.

My first step, in Spring 1990, was to invite local GPs to lunch in order to discuss my idea. To my joy they were very keen and wanted me to start immediately.

However, I had to stress that I needed at least three months to raise the necessary funds to employ qualified nurses.

I set an initial goal of £3,000 – a guess, but it was a start, and I was helped enormously by the chairman and nursing co-ordinators of a similar scheme in Buckinghamshire.

Major fundraising events included a concert in the school hall, a talk on Chatsworth House, and two village lunches, one of which included family and friends from afar. I entertained American ramblers who gave generous donations and for twelve years, I baked and sold bread to my Broad Campden neighbours. A friend, who was a member of the Rotary Club, filled the town hall with residents, and I gave a talk about my project.

Other events took place within a seven-mile radius of Chipping Campden, producing generous donations and proceeds. A silent auction was organised by friends. Most of the events and talks were supported by raffles, for which local businesses donated generous prizes. Monies donated in memory of residents following their funerals, added greatly to the funds.

Throughout this time, I was overwhelmed by the support and enthusiasm of the local community. During this exciting and busy period of fundraising, the doctors set up a Board of Trustees, chairman and treasurer/secretary to help and advise on what was becoming a major project for the whole Chipping Campden area.

By late Autumn 1990 I had raised my target. My first patient was at Christmas that year. It was a very intensive case and at that stage, we had only two nurses in addition to myself. In January, I advertised and quickly recruited thirteen more nurses. All were fully trained and around half of them had palliative experience through careers as district nurses, health visitors or working in a hospice.

I was able to consult the surgeries in our area to locate the cases which most needed our help. I visited every local surgery to talk to the doctors and district nurses. I subsequently arranged a nursing schedule and happily included myself, particularly when we were short staffed. I was always prepared to step in.

I have set the scene for the launch of Campden Home Nursing. The next part is a record of a conversation I had with my son. I had just retired and was recovering in hospital following a knee operation. It offered a good opportunity to describe my experiences. Our son, Will, is a GP in London, and at the time of our conversations, he was working at St Joseph's Hospice and was therefore well placed to discuss care of the terminally ill. The record of our conversation is, I believe, worth setting out here in full, including reference to some nineteen cases out of the 380 I was involved with. There is some repetition of cases, from various angles. This has been allowed to remain.

Note: apart from in the first case described [see footnote p.15] some details of the patients and families involved have been changed to maintain anonymity.

In conversation

Conversations between Jecca and her son, Dr Will Brook
March 2005

Will: As a place to start, I would like to ask you about a memorable patient you nursed.

Jecca: One of the families that first comes to mind is a young mother, 32. She had two small children, a boy and a girl, aged 6 and 7; married and living in a beautiful house in Blockley our next-door village. She'd had cancer for about 18 months when I got involved. She had colon cancer. By the time Campden nurses became involved she was a very sick young lady but trying to carry on as normally as she could for the sake of her children and her husband. She had very supportive parents and in-laws who spent a lot of time with her, caring for the children.

We started off just going for one night a week, which gradually increased over time. We got to know her and her husband very well. We became very close to them.

As she approached her death, we reduced the nurses to a group of just three, so she didn't have too many different faces.

By now, she was in bed all the time, and on an increased dose of morphine to keep her pain under control, and therefore sleepier. But one of the things she said to us early on was, "Please, never shut my bedroom door. I want the children to feel that they can come in and out whenever they like." The nurses spent a lot of time with the children in her room, playing games and amusing them. They were very natural and easy, the way they ran in and out. Indeed, they did that right up until her death, which was in the night, with two of my nurses present. In the morning, her husband went to tell the children that their mummy had gone. The little girl chose to reflect alone, whilst the little boy went to stand at the foot of his mummy's bed to see her one last time. He was six. He felt he wanted to do that. We had a lovely Requiem Mass for her, with the father and the two little children standing by her coffin the whole service. It was very touching. She was young at just 32, and we were all very sad when the end came.

The support of the nurses allowed the family time to plan and to enjoy their remaining days together and gave the couple time to talk about what the future may hold after her death. We kept in close touch with the family. The children grew up, and their father eventually remarried. They have three children together and he is happy again.[1]

Will: And so how long were you nursing her?

Jecca: We nursed her for almost a month. We normally get involved with the families towards the last weeks of a patient's life.

Will: That's the policy?

Jecca: It is, but we have had patients we have looked after for longer than that. Indeed, we had one patient we looked after for four months. But she was terminal all that time. It was a very difficult case, and we put it to the Trustees. They

---

1 We are very grateful to Andy Doran and his son and daughter, Dominic and Fionnghuala for permission to share details of this case. Andy Doran, her husband recalled the following: "There was a phone call I overheard (it wasn't private) between your mother and some bigwig at Cheltenham Hospital who thought Josephine couldn't possibly get equal care at home as she could in his Cancer Ward. It was like a game of top trumps, everything he said he had Jecca had or had access to better, which is why my wife was allowed to die in peace at home."

agreed that, if the GP felt that this patient was terminal, we could look after her. That's rather an exceptional case. More likely, we looked after a family for ten to fourteen days. But we were with the young mother almost an entire month. The three of us who nursed her continued to go back and visit the husband and the children. Indeed, I am great friends with them all still, and see them in Campden a lot. It has been a lovely friendship.

Will: Can you please say a bit about how this story started, who initiated it, where the referrals came from and what was the family's attitude to your help? Then can you take us through a bit about what you did with her; what the level of nursing was; how that escalated, and how it changed in the very last stages?

Jecca: The district nurses had been visiting this young woman for about a year off and on to try and control her symptoms. We came in around a month before her death; initially we were asked to stay with her for one night, because her husband was so tired. Gradually we increased the nights, and finally we were going in every night and about three-quarters of every day to share in the care with her husband, who was trying to keep life as normal as possible for the children. The first week we were there she insisted on us dressing her in the day, helping her down the stairs; often we had to carry her down as she was so weak.

After the first week, she could no longer come downstairs, but we could still get her out of bed and into a chair, and she liked that. She felt she was being more normal for the children. Gradually that decreased, and the last ten days of her life she was in bed all the time. Gradually our nursing increased as she slept more and more, and her level of consciousness went down. She was completely unconscious for the last three days of her life, and then we gave intensive nursing, and this time with the help of the district nurses. The Macmillan nurse had been coming in to advise on pain control and that sort of thing, and there were regular visits from the GP. But really, towards the end, it was just intensive nursing.

Will: The way you describe it, it sounds like a death that was peaceful in the end, an ideal case for you, and you provided a tremendous service for someone in that situation. If things had not gone so to plan towards the end, if her symptoms had been just uncontrollable, what would have happened? Were there many scenarios where you had got someone to a very late stage in their illness and then things got out of hand and they had to go to Hospital?

Jecca: It never actually happened, although I recall an incident when I was asleep in bed – it was midnight – and a GP had been called out to a patient of ours who we had just started nursing. Very quickly, the patient had begun to deteriorate, and the GP was called out. His pain was uncontrolled. The doctor asked me to go back to the house as the wife couldn't possibly spend the rest of the night alone. So, out I went. The GP was also present, and I have never in my life given anybody so much medication without it having an effect.

Finally, by the morning we got it under control, but I found that a very traumatic experience, and so did the GP. We met the next day, this GP and I, and another partner, and one or two of the nurses, and we worked through it.

In the case of the young mother, although it was very sad because she was so young, she did have a wonderful death. Her pain was completely controlled, she was at peace, life did go on fairly normally for their two children, and her husband said to me at the time, "If it had to be, then I don't think she could have had a better death." When we get involved we know we are not going to make the patients better, so our aim is to make the death as good as possible.

The case of the patient with the uncontrollable pain was difficult, because it was still relatively early days in the progression of their condition, which is probably why it was more distressing. But as time passed, the pain control got better and better. I did finally get to the stage of feeling that if we had a death that was full of pain and distress and agitation, we had failed somewhere, because the choice of drugs was so enormous that it was just a question of getting the cocktail right and experimenting a little. Most of the GPs I worked for were becoming more experienced with dosage because an increasing number of their patients stayed at home rather than go to hospital.

But to go back to what you said about having to put them in hospital because the pain was uncontrollable, we never had such an incident. In fourteen years we had only one patient who asked to go to a hospital and one to a hospice. The lady who wanted to go to hospice had a particularly distressing cancer and she had appalling breathing problems. Her husband found the process immensely difficult. She just said to me one day,

"I cannot die like this." We offered her a place at a hospice. It was a new hospice that was just opening and the nursing director turned out to be a colleague of mine who I'd met when I was training. This was a Saturday, and on the Monday the beds were being opened for the first time, and my patient was welcomed. She went up on the Monday and died on the Tuesday, but I saw her before her death and agreed she was in the right place. She felt loved and cared for there, and in the end, she had a peaceful death.

The other case was a gentleman with advanced cancer who wanted to go to hospital – I was with him at the time, and it was very late at night. I had just settled him in bed when he became very distressed; at first, we couldn't understand what it was. It wasn't pain. Finally, he said, "I want to go to the hospital; I will feel safe there." In the end I took him in my car and settled him in.

We took him to the cottage hospital where they were very sweet and welcomed him, and he died the next day. The sadness was that he and his wife had never been apart for one night of their lives; being apart was very traumatic. We spent a lot of time with his wife afterwards and visited her regularly. It was quite difficult for her, because she felt it was her fault that he had to go in, but it wasn't at all.

But those were the only two, out of almost 400 patients, that preferred a hospital environment rather than to be nursed at home.

Its also true that on a few occasions some people never made it home from hospital; even when we'd had a referral, which was a sad turn of events

But one case I remember very well of a young woman in hospital who had a very aggressive kind of tumour; she had a charming husband and a little boy of six. Her wider family was also involved – her parents also wanted her at home because they felt it was right that she died with the family together. I was asked to go to a case conference in the hospital, which I did. But first, I went in to see the lady herself. She couldn't speak, couldn't recognise anybody, was very restless and agitated. She was barely conscious. My concern was that we wouldn't get her home in time. But, I assured her husband and mother that, as far as we were concerned, I was prepared to try and get her home, although we warned the family that she might well die in the ambulance, she was so poorly. They were absolutely determined we should try. We arranged it and I organised my nurses to provide a full time rota because the patient was so ill. We got her home and settled her into bed; she lived for two hours. And of course, we were pleased on the one hand that we had just managed to get her back to her family, but sad that she had so little time with them. She had a completely peaceful death. The husband and the mother were unbelievably grateful to us, for pushing it. The hospital had said over and over, very caringly, she is just too ill to move.

We took the risk to fulfil their wish and it worked. In a way, it was an amazing stroke of luck with that patient, that it went just right, to have made it home.

Will: We had a situation not very dissimilar when I recently started at St Joseph's, and the luck went the other way. It wasn't our decision. The patient was coming from a hospital across town, over to East London. He died en route and his last moments on earth were in an ambulance, sitting in traffic. It was nobody's fault; everyone was trying to do the best thing. As I was the person receiving him at the other end, I felt badly for him and part of me thought somebody the other end should have just made a different decision (a bit like the doctor was saying in your case that she is too ill to be moved; I am sorry but events have overtaken us). Important to say though that decision making in medicine is always easy with hindsight.

Jecca: That might well have happened with us. Moving her into the ambulance, might have killed her. But I think what pleased me most was the reaction of her mother and husband. They were just so thankful and said, "If we just got her into the house alive, that would have been enough for us."

But that reminds me of another case, a young man with AIDS who was just a mile outside our area. He'd moved away from his family for many years. When he became ill, he tried getting in touch with his parents again; at this point he was clearly dying of AIDS, and they wanted him home. And because the circumstances were rather unusual, I asked my Trustees whether we could make an exception and nurse him outside our area, and they agreed that we could. We had it all set up, but he died on the way home. That made me feel very sad because, rather like you just said, they had been parted for so long, and the parents felt that the final thing they could do for him was to nurse him at home. But on the other hand, they were very understanding and realised that, as in your case, it was just very unfortunate, it was left too late.

In a way, in all those situations, even though the arrangement doesn't work out, there will still have been benefit because, in a sense, the parents will have been offered that act of kindness or that act of possibility for it to happen, and will have been left with that. Well, who knows what they would have been left with? I think it was as much a problem for us as perhaps it was for the parents. They were very generous to us about it. How can you tell? Nurses and doctors aren't gods. You can't predict exactly. But that saddens me as well though. But one hopes that generosity on the part of Campden Home Nursing was a help.

A rather nice thing happened over that case. I had never discussed with the nurses about looking after somebody with AIDS. It was a relatively new disease and there was some degree of fear surrounding it. I wrote to them all in confidence to ask if they had any qualms and without exception they all wrote back saying: "We don't know why you asked us." That was very nice.

Will: Lots of things come up as you start to talk about patients. When you say the operation has been going for fifteen years now, very few had to go back to hospital or hospice; what an amazing vindication not just of your local operation but of that as a model of care. In other words, you as a nurse-led plus GP service, can cope with very severe, very advanced illness at home. And it makes me think that, if this service was available everywhere, that aspect of hospices as provider of beds, becomes less crucial.

Jecca: I have very strong feelings about that. I do recognise the value of our scheme, and the other schemes now that have evolved in England. But I always felt the real way forward is for each hospice to have a home care team. Now, a lot of them do have home care teams, but they don't go in and nurse. They are more like Macmillan nurses. If every hospice had a team of nurses like mine, going in to actually to do the nursing and keep patients at home, the hospices would be less busy, less pushed for beds and so forth, it would save them a lot of time, and a lot of money. And then the need for schemes like mine wouldn't be there in the same way. It hasn't caught on.

A new hospice opened a few years ago just outside Stratford-on-Avon, and the head fund-raiser asked me to go and have lunch with him, to see the newly opened hospice, which I did. I was very impressed, and I met a lot of the staff and the nursing co-ordinator. It was all very exciting. And then he took me out to lunch and he started talking about raising millions to build a wing of beds. I said, "Before you start raising the millions, would you think of starting a scheme like mine?" And I am glad to say that is exactly the way they have gone. In fact, one of my nurses works for them and goes out into the community. I would never say there is not a need to have hospices with beds. But I am delighted that they have moved forward with home nursing. Maybe in time they will have beds too. But I am sure the way forward for hospices is to have a team like mine to supplement their services.

Will: Absolutely right and, in a way, the reason why I am keen for you to talk about what you have done is because it is so manifestly successful, and a very good solution to this problem. These things are of course complex but it's clearly more cost effective than hospices with bricks and mortar and beds, and so forth. You can deliver just as much expertise in that way. One imagines that, if this service was more available, more and more people would choose to die at home. What is skewed for me is that I work in a residential unit in a hospice;

many of the people who die there want to die in a hospice. There are all sorts of services like Macmillan nurses, our community palliative care teams, but there aren't services like your own. At some point in the future people are going to wake up to this, and so are funders. The amazing thing about your service is that it has never taken any public money – an extraordinary fact – although the quality of the care you provide has been very high from the start.

Jecca: One other thing I would say about that is that if the hospices had a home nursing service, you would have much easier access to the hospice.

There have been times with patients when I would have loved them to have gone in to have had intensive pain control – just for a couple of days, because there were times when we had five or six families to look after all at once. Therefore, we couldn't give them full 24-hour nursing because we didn't have enough nurses. I wouldn't say that the hospices weren't very co-operative, but we didn't have that close a link. Whereas if the nurses came from the hospices, there would be constant communication between the hospice and them. I just wonder whether that wouldn't make an even better service.

Will: Well the brilliant thing you have done is to get it off the ground, got it working, got it established. You have had some medical input, but I think I'm right in saying, very little specialist palliative care input. Essentially it's a nurse plus GP service providing palliative care. If for the next five or ten years there is always going to be a shortage of palliative care specialists and, probably, hospices, yours as a model of to how to organise services is just unbeatable.

Jecca: I think what I would say now is that, when I started, yes, I was a nurse. I did have some experience of palliative care but I needed to get much more up to date. The GPs I worked with had a certain amount of palliative care experience. But, overall, before I started, patients went to hospital or a hospice at the end of their lives. So, it was a very growing period, those 14 or 15 years.

I can count on one hand the number of times we had to consult a palliative consultant because, through publications, the GPs were keeping more up to date. They got to know more about it, and learned through experience – of course we were learning on the job all the time. A very crucial link here was the district nurses. I think I was very fortunate. I worked with 16 or 17 district nurses, and overall, because they had our support, they got keener on palliative care. Before we were around, they couldn't keep all those patients at home because they just didn't have the time. When we were established and could go in and take over from them, we all learned together along the route. And yes, sometimes, we did consult the pain control clinics. And, indeed, halfway through my time with the Trust, one of my GPs became the first palliative consultant in Cheltenham. I knew him personally very well, and now and again I did ask for his advice if we really got stuck, and he was always happy to help.

When I had lectures for the nurses in our house, he very often came and brought us up to date. But it was big learning experience for the GPs, the district nurses and ourselves.

Will: Can you give me any other examples of specific situations where you got stuck?

Jecca: There were occasions. One example I had was a relatively young woman who had advanced cancer. She had a lot of anger about her illness. Although she had good care from the GP and the district nurses and subsequently our nurses, she refused all pain control. Her pain became quite unbearable, but she wouldn't accept anything from the GP or the district nurses. So, we got onto Michael Sobell Hospice and one of their specialists, an expert on pain control, very kindly agreed to come out to this woman's house. He came and spent a long time with her. We were there, and the district nurse was there, and we all talked together about it. Sadly, by the end of his visit she was still refusing to have pain control.

Will: Why was she so adamant about this?

Jecca: I and the GP talked a lot about this together alone, and we concluded that she was someone who had always been very much in control of her life, of her work, of her family. And by taking strong pain relief she felt she was losing control, and wouldn't be as alert as she would have been without it – even though the pain became so unbearable. We just couldn't think of any other explanation of why she behaved like that. Sadly, it was undeniably a very difficult last chapter of her life.

Will: In hindsight, how could things have been different? With a patient like that, there is a limit beyond which you cannot cross, you clearly cannot insist that the patient follows your agenda. Was there anything else that might have been done?

Jecca: We covered every option with her. We suggested that she might go into the hospice under this specialist who would personally monitor her care and her pain control. He is a man who has a wonderful, gentle way with the patients, and we felt sure that she would be persuaded. But she declined. So, unfortunately, this colleague left feeling as we did, very frustrated that we were unable to do more for this patient, because our job wasn't to take the control out of our patients' hands.

Will: On this theme of how often you needed specialist services, can you give me a very rough breakdown in figures over fourteen years? What I'd like to know is roughly what percentage had a lot of GP input and what percentage had hospice and specialist palliative care input?

Jecca: That's interesting, because the numbers are not as I would have expected them to be. In fourteen and a half years I looked after almost 400 families. I worked with 17 GPs – of course, they all varied tremendously. But what did surprise me was how rarely we had to seek further advice. The former GP colleague I mentioned in Cheltenham who was a palliative consultant and whom I knew I could ring at any time was consulted only three times. The patient I have just talked about was the only time we got the Palliative Consultant involved substantially. But what I did do on occasion, was call on my colleagues who ran similar schemes, to ask their advice, and very often that's all I needed. The numbers were surprisingly low when we had to go further than the GP.

Will: Can you give me a rough percentage?

Jecca: When I started the Trust, we had twelve patients in the year. Gradually, that built up slowly, and I think the most we ever had was 45 in a year. But it used to average out at around 35 patients a year. I would think we only asked for hospice advice once or twice a year at the most. The longer we were going, the more doctors got involved in the palliative side – in a way through us I suppose. Whereas before, they sent so many patients to a hospital or a hospice because we weren't there.

Will: In order to have that link, was it effectively a sort of informal colleague-to-colleague way of speaking to someone because you happened to know the palliative care consultant? It sounds like there wasn't any formal channel of communication between you and the hospice.

Jecca: The Trust paid all my nurses to do a minimum of three education days a year, and more if they wished. A lot of these took place in St Richard's Hospice, which was a day hospice in

Worcester. We had an extremely high standard of lecturers there. And very often, after one of these sessions, I would speak with them at the end or write to them, and many of them came down to my monthly nurses' evenings to give us a talk on their specialty. These were all hospice-based specialists. We had doctors, nurses, physiotherapists, music therapists, psychotherapists, alternative medicine therapists, and so on, but they were all people who were working with the dying. Over the years we had six lectures a year for 14 years. We had a lot of lectures, all pertaining to palliative care.

Will: In terms of getting advice, the link was informal?

Jecca: Indeed. What I could do, which I did sometimes, was to ring St Richard's Hospice, present them with a problem, and ask their advice as to which channel I should go down. And sometimes it wasn't necessarily the palliative consultant. They were extremely helpful. But no, we didn't have a strict formal relationship. If you are talking about numbers, we did it rarely. My feeling was that, the longer I was doing it and got more experienced, so too did the GPs, because a lot of them hadn't had a service that allowed people to die at home at all. By the time I retired a lot of them were very interested and very experienced in it.

Will: It is interesting how almost completely self-sufficient a service you were, along with local GPs. It is striking how little specialist medical input you needed.

Jecca: Yes, I think that side surprised me, really. But, again, through our experience and therefore the district nurses having more experience of keeping their patients at home, it was a tremendous learning curve we all experienced together. By the time I left, most of my district nurses, of which there were then 17, were very knowledgeable in palliative care. In a sense, one of the strengths of the Trust was that we were so self-sufficient. Even regarding GPs, it was very seldom that we had to call them out at night and so on. They would visit in the day in the normal way, but we managed very well on our own.

***

Will: A slightly different subject now. I want to ask about the 'model' of palliative care: the course it usually takes, in a way such that hospices can best operate. It tends to be centred around cancer as a diagnosis. Sometimes from our point of view, it feels like you have this wonderful world of palliative care, but the passageway into it is narrow. If you fit the bill age-wise and in terms of diagnosis, then you can make your way through that gate and you can enter this place and get very good care. However, if you don't tick those boxes, if someone has had a very severe stroke or if you have severe emphysema, or heart failure, often there isn't such a good fit. This is a little simplistic, and isn't a critique of what goes on in hospices, but I am just interested if you have thoughts about how the ideas of the hospice/palliative care movement could penetrate a wider array of non cancer illness at the end of life?

Jecca: Yes, I was very much aware when I was working, that if you had a patient who had, if you like, a straightforward cancer, and then a secondary cancer and clearly in the terminal stage, the whole process of the disease was much more easily diagnosed and you could more accurately give a time limit in the sense that we came in towards the end of somebody's life. You could gauge that accurately. But, as soon as you get into heart disease, as you say, or chronic disease of any sort, it is very difficult.

We did have a patient who had a chronic neurological condition to some extent but who had a lot of other things wrong, and in the end, cancer too. Her GP said it was a terminal case and we moved in and provided care, and four months later, we were still there. The Trust was fine about that because the GP said the stage was terminal. But I think you run into that sort of case more with the chronically sick. A good example is motor neurone disease, where the end sometimes goes on for a very long time, and it's hard to know at what stage to get involved. I think if somebody has secondary cancer, it is much easier to encompass them in palliative care rather than chronic, very slow, progressive illness. Of course, they need the care just as much as anybody else does, but it is a very difficult decision. If we went in when we felt we should go in, we would be looking after them for months and months, and then you face the risk of running out of nurses. It is something that has always worried me, because I feel that the area of care of the chronically sick is still very 'grey'.

I feel that, with the progress of hospice at home groups, this is something that should be addressed, because their needs are long-term and therefore in some ways greater.

Will: What's interesting here is that the research that has been done on doctors' accuracy of predicting prognosis suggests that they aren't very good at it; that is, predicting the 'remaining time'. If your rule is that you are basically geared up to going in for the last month of life, I am amazed you could get it right so often, because certainly in the hospice we are always caught out; often either patients die much sooner or they die later than predicted.

Jecca: Yes, I am surprised we didn't run into difficulties more often. Occasionally we were asked to get involved much too soon. I had a case once where I had a letter from a GP, which was unusual because I had all my referrals from the district nurses. He said he had a couple; the gentleman was dying and they needed help now. This was the number. Perhaps foolishly, I didn't go through the district nurse, I went directly to see the family, and the gentleman concerned was up and dressed and opened the door to me.

Once inside, I discovered his wife was very frail following a stroke. And yes, he was having difficulty looking after her, but the GP indicated to me that he was the one that was dying, and he clearly wasn't in the terminal phase of his illness.

That presented us with a problem. Because of the nature of our work I couldn't just walk out on this family, so we provided them with two nights of nursing. Meanwhile, the family got some help from social services. He did in fact die fairly soon after. It was a complicated case with some unexpected twists and turns. The unusual referral process was a difficulty, but I got wise to this, and I would always go back through the district nurse. I suppose it was rather extraordinary, but so rarely were we caught out. I think in all the time I was running Campden Home Nursing, I only had to go back to the Trustees three times to ask them whether we could prolong care for a month. And of course, they never quibbled with these requests because they believed that if the GP confirmed the case was terminal, that was fine with them.

Will: So is it the case in a situation like that where it was a grey area in terms of whether the diagnosis was entirely suitable for you, or the stage of the illness was entirely suitable, your team would go in as a sort of holding strategy? Did that sometimes happen?

Jecca: Yes. On one occasion we had a case conference with the district nurses and the relatives, and we explained that in fact our job wasn't to look after a spouse in a household who had frailties but no terminal illness. But, because the family member who was our patient was obviously ill (albeit less frail) we weren't going to just walk out and leave the family. We gave them two days' grace, and again, we went back to the Trustees and discussed the case with them, and that was fine with them. But that only happened once, getting as far as that, because I learned from experience, and instead I would talk to the GP concerned directly, and say, "I discussed this with the district nurses and they don't feel that the family is ready for us yet. Maybe they need some input from social services." But, as I said, this only happened once.

Will: If we just think further about applying the ideas of the palliative care improvement to different scenarios, given that Campden Home Nursing is providing a very specific service, which is sending nurses into homes to do nursing care, I completely accept that model of care doesn't obviously extend itself to, say, Alzheimer's. Terminal care in Alzheimer's is a complicated area: more complex issues about prognosis and long-term degeneration, and a different sort of care. It brings up the notion of end of life needs of very elderly people who may less often fall into the palliative care category. Is it not the case that the ideas of Cicely Saunders and other pioneers of palliative care need very much to be extended to those groups – even if the problems are so much more long-term and more complex?

Jecca: Very much so. Palliative care is palliative care, whatever the patient is dying of. I think the difficulty is, which we experienced when I started, if I had too many patients at any one time, it is very difficult to provide enough care for everybody. Obviously, I had a limited number of nurses, and I had to take into consideration that if I had as many as, say, 30 nurses, most of the time I wouldn't be able to use them at all, because we wouldn't have enough patients. Therefore, we ran at about 16 or 17 nurses, because overall it was enough to give that care package for that family. When you run into people with Alzheimer's or a chronic disease that goes on for a long time, I think it's a completely different concept, and it would be lovely to feel that they had the sort of care that we could give our families, because terminal care is terminal care, and their need is enormous, doubly so because of their mental frailty. However, I think it's something completely different that must be addressed because of resources and because of the number of nurses. Therefore, I think, so many of these patients go into homes, because they can be cared for collectively in a sense, because their needs are different. That isn't necessarily the right care for them, but I think, as things stand, there isn't the facility for trusts like ours to look after such long-term patients. This is a very grey area that needs to be addressed. But trying to find the answer is a difficult one.

Will: One thing I immediately think of when you mention nursing homes is that you have experience of actually working in them when I was a young boy, in the 1970s. Let me ask specifically about that period – 1972/73. I am sure there must have been all sorts of 'end of life' care situations that arose then. I am interested in this different era, a generation ago, and in a very different setting. How good was the palliative care, and then how good was the terminal care?

Jecca: Well, I think I was lucky, because I worked in a nursing home with 25 rooms, and we had one GP who looked after all the patients. He used to say that there comes a point in everybody's life when the quality of their life is unacceptable, and he would be ready to increase the drugs they were on for pain control, and we were all made very aware of the fact that, given that increase of drugs, that may well have hastened the end of life, and we were very open with the families about this. I do remember one case of a son saying that, so long as his father was comfortable, under no circumstances did he want his drugs increased, and we respected that. But, overall, the patients either had nobody or elderly relatives, or children who understood that the quality of their loved ones' lives was very poor. I think in this case I was very fortunate in having a GP who didn't feel that to preserve life at any cost was the right thing to do. His emphasis was on quality of life.

Will: And so would you and your nursing colleagues have felt this was a humane place? How would this sort of nursing home and the care you were providing stand up to scrutiny today, when it's a more public issue?

Jecca: We had an excellent matron, who was experienced in palliative care, because none of our patients went out of the nursing home; eventually they all died there. I do wonder whether we could have given the same care package. I think there was more freedom then than there is now, and my feeling is that today, not just because people live longer, I think people strive to keep the sick alive for much longer now than they did in the past. I don't have that much to compare it with, but my feeling is that, knowing how the different rules and regulations changed over the 14 years that I was nursing, how much more regulated everything is now.

Will: When you say 'freedom', you have alluded to something which is about the attitude of your GP, around quality of life and so forth, but what do you mean?

Jecca: I can just think of one example when I was doing nights in the nursing home. There was always plenty of medication should we need to give it during the night and, obviously, even in those days, we had to get the doctor's permission, but it meant that he didn't have to leave his house and come back to the home.

One of the things we found difficult through these 14 years of Campden Home Nursing, and this is where the GPs varied so much, quite a number of them wouldn't allow us to have extra medication in the house, so that sometimes, especially late at night, we had to call them out, quite unnecessarily in my opinion, simply to prescribe and increase the morphine. We had an arrangement with some GPs that we could give on the basis of a verbal request over the phone. Then in the morning, on the doctor's first visit, he or she would sign for it. And, because of that, I saved the doctors coming out many times. And, in quite a lot of cases, we had the permission to use our discretion, so often, even these late night phone calls were unnecessary. This system worked in the patients' benefit, because it meant we didn't have to delay treatment and we could save the patient from unnecessary pain.

Will: Extending it further back, when you finished training in the early '60s, do you have a sense of what attitudes were like to terminal care then, at the start of your career?

Jecca: For a period of my training I worked in a brain hospital where, on the whole, the patients were critically ill. We had a great number of unconscious patients, either post-accident or post-surgery. Therefore, we lost a lot of patients, and I think that was when I really took the problems of death on board. I suppose I was 18 years old at the time, and hadn't had an awful lot of experience of patients dying; obviously some, but on the whole, these cases were handled by the Sister and the senior staff nurses. But in the brain hospital we all had to get involved. It used to bother me a little that the patients didn't seem to have enough care, but as a young woman I didn't feel that we cared enough for the families. In recent years this extended care has been an enormous part of running the Trust; I would say more than 50% of the care is for the families involved. When we went into a family where the patient was already in a coma, they would get all the nursing care they needed, but there is only a certain amount you can do for somebody with that degree of illness. Therefore maybe 70 or 75% of our time would have been looking after the families.

Will: Picking up on one thing you said when you were talking earlier, the way you described the work in an individual case, you described it as 'one of our families' instead of 'one of our patients', as if almost primarily you were looking after families rather than looking after patients. Just say a little bit more about this.

Jecca: I think the reason I said that is because when we go into a house, the package is the patient, the families, the dogs, and whoever else lives there. One is embracing the whole unit. It may be a patient and friends because they have no family. But you don't just take on the patient.

So, the package from our point of view is their whole package, which is the entire family. One of our jobs is to get into their day to day lives in the easiest possible way so that we then become part of things – just an extended member of the family. So, the emphasis is on the family.

Will: I am interested in the spread of time scales, because you have been a nurse for a long time – even though it was later in your career that you got interested in palliative care. I want to ask you a bit about your career in relation to that. Let me start with a 'fantasy scenario' – the thing that didn't happen. Let's say, throughout your married life, you stayed working. Let's say you stayed in nursing; you had gone on up through the ranks. You had either become a senior district nurse or a senior matron in a hospital. Do you think your interests and ideas and focus would have turned to palliative care in the way that it did?

Jecca: I often wonder what path I would have taken had I stayed in nursing. In the 1970s I decided to do my first bereavement course; even then it was something that had been on my mind for a long time. Without thinking so much of palliative care, I was very interested in bereavement, and did quite a lot of work with the bereaved. Ending up in palliative care just seemed to be a natural way forward. I had some experience in the 1980s of looking after one or two patients who were dying. So that added to my interest in it, alongside the bereavement care. It was then influenced by caring for both my parents some years apart. That had a terrific effect on me, and I found it a wonderfully fulfilling experience. If I hadn't had that experience it's difficult to say whether I would have ended up in palliative care. That was a very strong factor.

Will: Why did you do a bereavement course in the 1970s?

Jecca: We were living in London and I was doing a bit of locum nursing. I talked to several friends who were doing bereavement care, and I had always found that I was comfortable with grieving people, although at that stage I had no experience and no training. A lot of people are not at ease with the bereaved, and I felt I was, and I felt it was a way forward for me.

Will: And this was before your mum died?

Jecca: My mother died in 1976, and my first course – I did one before she died – I think it was in the early 1970s, and then I did a much longer one in 1979 when we were back in London. That was a much more in-depth course under the umbrella of CRUSE Bereavement Care and it was at a time when I was reading a lot about bereavement and palliative care. And particularly after looking after my mother, I think the seed was already sown; I just wanted to learn more and more about it.

Will: Caring for your mother – was that the first time you had looked after a dying person in a very concerted way?

Jecca: Yes, it was certainly the first time I had looked after somebody in their own home, and it turned out to be for seven months. I would have been living with her anyway at that stage because we had no house of our own, moving round in the Royal Air Force for my husband, David's, job. It just felt like a very natural place for me to be, being the only nurse in the family. I had the time to do it, and it was a wonderful experience.

Will: I had forgotten that you were living with her anyway; there was a sort of symmetry to it. But had you not been living with her; would you have felt able to get as involved so easily? Would you have just offered your services and got involved? Or was it something that just came about almost by default?

Jecca: I think what was made easy for me was because we were in a period of service life where

David had to attend courses before he took up a big command job, and I had no home. I would have gone to live with my mother anyway. In a sense you can say it was just meant to be. I have often thought how it would have been had she been diagnosed terminally ill in the summer of 1976, and we had been posted to Germany or somewhere else in the UK even. I suppose the answer to that is, I would have spent quite a lot of that time looking after her. I was never presented with the dilemma of wanting to be with the family or with my mother. In a way the decision had been made for me.

Will: What about that home setting? You describe a scenario many, many people find themselves in; they are at home, illness enters the family, and they have to take it on board. You are unusual in that you are a nurse. What about the scenario where you happened to be living with your mum? I am sure there were all sorts of things going on between you and a sense of starting to help her take on board this thing that was happening. What about when your involvement crossed over into nursing care and you were doing physical nursing? Was that a difficult decision? Was it difficult to do? Did it change the atmosphere in the house? What was that like?

Jecca: This was something I used to think about a lot, wondering how easy it would be for me to do the more personal things for my mother. Fortunately for her, she maintained her dignity right to the end. Unfortunately, because of breathing problems she ended her days in hospital. But for the seven months that I had her at home, she was still able, right to the end, to attend to her personal needs, which was important for her. It wasn't a problem for me at all.

In the case of my father he needed much more help. When I arrived to look after him, I became a teacher to my stepmother. She was afraid of doing anything for him because he was so terribly ill. She was afraid of hurting him, and she had no experience of nursing. But over the six weeks I was there I was able to teach how to take on board some of the more intimate tasks for my father and, again, although it wouldn't have worried me at all, it never really occurred to me that I had to do those things because she was there. And I felt that was important to maintain that dignity for them both.

Will: Just going back to your mum, then. In your heart of hearts, would you have liked her to have remained at home, and for you to have cared for her until she died? When she went to hospital, was there a sense of disappointment, loss, somehow letting her down. Did you feel thwarted in some way?

Jecca: Towards the end she was having severe pain in her spine and, indeed, investigation showed that the cancer had spread. The GP who was delightful, very nice to my mum and myself and co-operative, suggested that we put her into hospital to get the pain under control. And when we took her in, I really felt this was what would be done, and I would have her back. I let her go into hospital knowing that she would come home to die because we had discussed it thoroughly together. When she went into hospital, she deteriorated very quickly, and her breathing became very difficult and laboured. Within twelve hours of being in hospital she was certainly still talking but she wasn't indicating that she wanted to go home in any way. It didn't come up, and I spent almost all the time with her. In fact, I think it was on the second night/third morning, early morning, she died. They gave her a room of her own and various of the family were with her. It was a peaceful death, and I don't think she was in the end stressed by not being at home. I did find it very hard because I'd had her at home for so long, and I felt I hadn't quite fulfilled my promise to her. But, as the years have gone by, I think now that she was content.

Will: Yes, it's interesting that there's a long passage of time, and there is a different perspective later. But I can well imagine that, having done so much, then somehow all the decision-making is taken out of your hands. In some cases that's a difficult moment.

Jecca: Yes, in one sense I did feel I was letting her down. I was proud of the fact that I had managed to keep her at home for that long. But I think through my experiences of running the Trust I can feel in my heart that what we did was right for her, looking back. But because of my emotional involvement, (very different to looking after all the families I had during those fourteen years) yes, it was a problem for me. But I think I can look back now and say it was right for her.

Will: I am interested in this, because I think issues about control and being the person making decisions, and somehow being 'in the driver's seat' either as the patient or as the carer, has all sorts of implications. I am interested to see if you have later stories or anecdotes about there being emotional issues between carers or between carers and families where it gets into slightly more complicated territory. Even for me now, working in the hospice, there are issues about who is making the decisions, ceding control, and the decision-making (whatever the situation is) being somehow taken away.

Given what you know now about looking after families and the complexities that go on in that setting, and the dynamics that there might be with the spouse, among the siblings, among more distant family members, do you have a perspective on that time? For each of these two important episodes, as you looked after both your parents. Looking back on those events, when you were much newer to palliative care, do you have a different 'take' on some of the issues that can arise within families at end of life?

Jecca: One big thing was that, of course, being my parents, I was totally emotionally involved. I was involved in the emotions of all my siblings, and those close to my parents. Later, during the years of the Trust, in the case of my families, yes, of course, I had my favourites – unspoken of because that's human nature. Some I got very close to, and it was more difficult. Overall, and I think this is partly to do with age, as well as how close one was to the families, one learns the discipline of standing back, taking a more objective view.

I learned this very early on in the hospice in Edinburgh. The way I dealt with not taking my work home was that when you have left the hospice or a patient's home, there is actually nothing more you can do for them. So, you leave it at the front door. And, in my case, running the Trust, I might have seen five families in one day; they aren't interested in the other families in your rotation. So, I had to leave each family at the door and pick up the next one. But I believe that's something that came with age and indeed now, if I was in a position where I was looking after either a sibling or a close relative or a very close friend, I may think differently again. With my parents I was totally involved, providing round the clock care, dealing with their emotions and the emotions of those round us in the family. But at work with my families, because you are coming into the situation so late in their lives, of course you get involved (otherwise you shouldn't be doing the job), but you do also have a capacity for objectivity. Getting very involved when you are there and on the job, but then standing back in between.

Will: In relation to your parents do you feel like there were any issues about you making decisions on their behalf, being so close to them? Not only being their daughter but being their carer as well? Can you get too close to a case like that?

Jecca: That's a difficult question to answer because I've only got two examples of that – my mother and my father. But I think, especially with my mother, I was in such close touch with my siblings all the time that I never felt that any decision I made (although they might have gone along with it) was ever made on my own. And in both cases I had very good back-up from not only family but the medical services as well. I was lucky there – excellent GPs in both cases, excellent district nurses, people I could always lean on and turn to.

Will: Regarding those experiences with your mother and your father, they were at different periods of your life, in different settings. I imagine it was very intense – looking after somebody dying as a nurse is in some ways more intense than as a doctor – because you're there with them 24/7. Emotionally, these were very big situations to have to take on board. Have you been able to translate these experiences into your subsequent working life and care work? Or, is it the case that because you were so close to them, they were just an entirely different category of situation?

Jecca: I don't really feel that. What I do feel is that I was extremely lucky with the relationship I had with my mother and my father. Therefore, there was never any decision about whether I wanted to go and look after them. I loved them both deeply, and it seemed a completely natural thing to do.

Although the two scenarios were different, I look back now and I feel sure that the Trust was the result of looking after them. Whether or not I would have started the Trust without the parental experience, I don't know, but I feel that was it, especially after I had looked after my father and we were coming up to leaving the Royal Air Force. I had known for some time that I very much wanted to do something for myself, and something on my own. And it just seemed a natural way forward, after having those two very special experiences.

Will: So, your father died in 1989, shortly before Dad left the RAF; in those terms, the time was right. But give me a sense of what those personal projects may have been had it not been starting Campden Home Nursing? Then, just take us through a bit about moving to Gloucestershire and how things moved on after that.

Jecca: I spent a lot of time between March and July of 1989 (during which time we left the

RAF) thinking to myself, if I could provide end-of-life care for my parents, surely I might be able to extend this service to my community. The feeling wouldn't leave me. But I don't think I had the confidence to express it so clearly at the time. It was only after a lunch date with two of our local GPs in Gloucestershire, that the idea took solid shape. One of them just happened to say, "What are you going to do with your energy now you have come to live here?" and the idea just fell into place. We went on from there. It just seemed a natural progression that had been very strongly in my mind. Whether or not I would be able to fulfil it, I had no idea, but I was determined to try.

Once I had really got the idea into my head that this perhaps was something I could take forward I looked at both scenarios: looking after long-term patients, and then palliative care. I was just overwhelmingly drawn towards palliative care. I also felt there were a lot of people in the nursing world who were already caring for long-term patients, and when I started there were, perhaps, not enough looking after the strictly palliative care patients in the home. I quickly realised that it was going to be a challenge, to gather a team of nurses.

Will: The speed with which you recruited 13 nurses is amazing. One potential constraint on your service growing must have been nurse recruitment. What is amazing in Gloucestershire, there's a sense that this was the right charity at the right time in the right place. So, on that very practical front, while Gloucestershire is quite an affluent county does it just happen to have a lot of nurses around?

Jecca: I just think we were very fortunate. We took on all of those 13 nurses. We were incredibly lucky to be starting such a trust in Gloucestershire. I think it would have been very different in a city. We were also fortunate with the calibre of our nurses. Having helped with launching three other similar groups, some of them had great difficulty getting nurses. In our case I think a lot of it was luck.

And these were nurses who were working part-time, or some had full-time jobs, some retired, some had taken a career break. Something I would say was that, when I went round talking about the Trust to groups, quite a lot of ex-nurses were there, and I would say probably nearly half of the nurses I recruited had retired from being district nurses or health visitors or hospice nurses, and hadn't really thought about coming back into nursing. When they realised they could come back in and do the nursing they loved most, but on their terms, for as little or as much as they wanted, they found that a very attractive proposition. I think that was one of the reasons we sourced so many nurses from the retired. And some of those nurses went on nursing to their early 70s.

Will: The amazing thing is it sounds like within a month of starting, you had not far off a full complement of team members?

Jecca: It sounds very quick, but I think our luck was having selected such an outstanding Board of Trustees. This meant I was released from all administrative responsibilities, aside from recruiting nurses and setting up the nursing care. And that was the case for the fourteen years I ran the Trust. We obviously had changes in the key positions. The Treasurer, the Chairman changed over the years, but they were always of excellent calibre. This meant I never had to worry about that side of things. We had some periods when we were a little low on nurses, a little bit more difficult to recruit them, but, generally, during this period, we were never in a position whereby we couldn't fulfil a family's needs.

Will: So, just to be clear, your area was a seven-mile radius – about 150 square miles. What was the population?

Jecca: That's difficult to answer, but we said we would care for any terminally ill patient within that area, whichever doctor was looking after them. In other words, we didn't go as far as Stratford-Upon-Avon. But if the doctors had a patient within our area, we would look after them. It's difficult to put an exact number on it; we managed around 35 to 37 patients a year. This is guess work, but let's say we're looking at a population of maybe 9,000 people.

Will: One other intriguing thing is that you settled on the size of the operation, and perhaps with an element of luck, you managed to recruit just the right number of people. And it seems to be a good size, because it wasn't too mammoth an administrative burden for one person, and it meant it was very local in its emphasis.

Jecca: I feel very strongly about that, because over the years as we became financially stable, there were people on the outside urging us to grow, and I always said, and indeed my partner agreed with me, that the strength of our group was its size. I should mention here that after six years on my own, I realised that I could not manage without a co-ordinator. Fortunately, Arlette Gaskell was already part of my team. She had worked without a break all her life and she agreed to share the job with me, working one month on, and one month off. This allowed me to have a break and it suited her. We formed a close friendship. Furthermore, she was always there, and her wide experience and advice was enormously helpful. The group was small, it was personal, and it never got out of our control. But I feel that, had we been any bigger, we would have had to have more coordinators and it wouldn't have been nearly so personal. Some of the other groups have grown very large, and I dare say they have found ways of managing. But I think, and I am glad to say my successor agrees, that one of our main strengths is our size, and that it's very workable. It's never beyond our control. I think that's a very important part of it.

Will: In organizational and political terms, what's very striking is that it's a community very much helping itself. In terms of finances, much of the organizational work is done on a voluntary basis: the Board of Trustees is not paid at all. And at the start you, and later Arlette, as co-coordinators, were on a relatively low wage, which is something to come back to. Of course your nurses were paid at the full rate from the beginning. Financially, it is an operation that is self-sustaining, and one could say that is tied up in it being such a local entity. The trust can inspire loyalty and therefore raise funds, and maintain goodwill for it, because it remains so local.

Jecca: That is true, and when I go about my retired life now, I often meet people who have been touched by the Trust. Perhaps we haven't looked after their husband or wife or child, but a friend of a friend or a relation. And then offshoots of it have been fantastic for fundraising. We have had a considerable number of people approaching their Golden Weddings insisting that instead of presents, they would like to see donations go to the Trust, which is very touching. And that also spreads the news.

I get a lot of calls from outside our area asking me if there is such a scheme in other parts of the country. Indeed, there are, but not, of course, anything like enough. And there are large areas of England which don't have any such service at all.

Will: On that subject of raising money, you do have an inbuilt advantage of the charity being what it is, in as much as things surrounding care of the dying do seem to be able to raise money through donations. As an aside, we had a conversation at the hospice recently where I was just playing devil's advocate and was saying how for many people the prospect of dealing with a hospice is quite frightening, as though hospice care always relates to end of life; I asked if there was a case for the whole palliative care movement to re-brand itself; to come up with a different word for 'hospice'? Dr Hillier, our director, said that, in some ways yes, you could argue that. But one of the cases for not doing that is that hospice as a word has this almost magical ability to raise funds.

Jecca: Hospices are not necessarily for dying in. A crisis during the terminally ill stage may involve time in the hospice, but patients often do come home to die.

I agree with you about raising funds. But I think – and this is the same with Macmillan nurses – if you ask the average man in the street what Macmillan nurses do, they would say they do what we do – which they don't. They do not do hands-on care, and funds are raised very easily for Macmillan. They get involved earlier, usually at the time of diagnosis and they give advice and are in touch with families.

Will: Back to the specifics of managing families, were there sometimes perhaps differences of opinion – some of the family wanting you, some other members of the family not wanting you?

Jecca: Just feeling rather possessive about the patient, realising that they couldn't actually cope with the whole thing, and yet resented our presence. On the other hand, usually, within a few hours of us being there, they came round. Especially after, say, they'd had us there for one night, and they'd had a good rest, and realised we weren't really a threat to them. I think some families felt threatened by us.

Will: In what ways?

Jecca: That we were going to take over, and they would no longer have any say in their loved ones' care. I always emphasised to the families that they were the boss. Alongside the district nurses, we were just there to help them in whatever way we could. I had a patient once – an elderly lady who was looked after by a younger relative. She was a difficult nursing case; she had a wound that wouldn't heal, and was doubly incontinent. Her relative was fantastic. I used to go every day, and I could see that things needed doing. But whenever I offered – perhaps to change the bed or the patient's nightdress – this family member would say, "No, no, it's fine. I'll do it when you've gone. Thank you for coming." When this old lady died, her relative had coped entirely alone. We never went in to do a nursing shift at all. I went on to see the family and said, "We didn't really do anything for you." And the response was "Well, you did, actually. You were at the end of the telephone all the time." And that made me realise from quite early on how valuable that was – that one of us was on the end of the telephone 24 hours a day.

Occasionally there were situations that had unexpected outcomes. We had one patient I remember where the house was small and space was a real issue. Quite a noisy environment. They were a family not very well resourced in a way, and yet amazingly resilient, and terribly supportive of each other. The patient was a young man dying of cancer.

We did fourteen nights in a row, and I had to find a different nurse each night. I went to the funeral service, to find hundreds of people packed into the church. I got a call about three weeks later from a young woman, one of the several children. She said: "Is that the nurse? You looked after my brother. Well, I want to meet you in town tomorrow." I said: "Well, actually I am working, but I could send one of my other nurses."

But no, it had to be me.

I had no idea who I was going to meet, and this very shy young woman came up holding a carrier bag which she duly handed over. Luckily, I didn't drop it, because it was full of money – over £400. They'd been raising money in their village for this boy. On the one hand, it was a difficult house to nurse in, although it was a very touching family. And then they did something like that. Despite their limited means, such generosity. It makes you remember what a privilege it is to do this work.

Will: What I wanted to ask you about scenarios where you get differences of opinion. Not so much between family members, because I imagine that's a bit more common. But where you get differences of what ought to happen between the family and the patient. I can think of it going both ways: either where one's inclination is to side with the family if one feels the patient is not of fully sound mind and not making entirely rational choices. Or sometimes the other way, because you feel the family has their motives distorted. I wonder if you can think of examples where, potentially, you are in the middle?

Jecca: When the patient becomes semi or unconscious, and therefore there isn't any dialogue anymore, at that stage the families can get very frightened. Therefore, they lean quite heavily on you. I would say that almost always, the families will take your advice – especially if you have consulted the doctor and district nurses and it has been a team decision. As far as possible we didn't go against the family's wishes, because we wanted them to feel that they were in charge. I remember very few instances whereby, with time and patience, and perhaps bringing in the GP and talking and going through it, they wouldn't come around.

One issue is difficult; stopping feeding. That's very final. On the other hand, it's very distressing to see a loved one choking or coughing terribly. You get to the stage where they can't swallow, and you must stop fluids. That can be very difficult for the families. But if you go on making them feel confident that you are doing the best for that person's comfort while they're dying, overall, they come round. There's an exception to all these rules, but on the whole, because you're the professional (in all honesty, often you don't have all the answers) just the fact that you are the nurse or the GP, they think you know everything and they'll abide by that. But it's always done with the family's consent.

Will: To specifics, then. If you've moved into the terminal phase and there is a decision to be made about the change in emphasis – for example, feeding is going to stop, fluids are going to stop, medication is going to be upped; would that be a nursing decision, or would that be in liaison with the GP?

Jecca: If it happened during the night I would (as I always did) ring the district nurses first thing so that when they came into the office, they have an up-to-date report. I would say to them, "I tried to give some oral medication in the night, and we had a lot of coughing and difficulty in swallowing." And then they would take it to the GP. He or she would then come out, then the district nurse would set up a syringe driver. Yes, it's a team effort.

Will: With the issue of being able to keep people at home at the end of life, one very specific thing that sometimes comes up is whether there is value in putting up a drip when somebody is dying, as symptom relief. A specific point – is it the case that you would never put up a subcutaneous drip in someone's house?

Jecca: We were not allowed to.

Will: So that isn't an option. In thinking about the last 48 hours of life, can you think of an example of having a patient where issues and decisions must be made? You're in quite a dynamic situation then where, maybe, all the treatment you are giving for symptomatic purposes must be upped and upped. We have mentioned how you would go about getting a syringe driver started. For instance, is it the case that a doctor would have a regimen of medications written up on an 'as needed' basis, and then it's at the nurses' discretion?

Jecca: Yes, but in the case of Campden Home Nursing, only if it was at night when it had already been discussed with the district nurses; if it was in the day, unless we had talked about it earlier, I would go through her again and say, "This is what we propose to do," and she would say, "That's fine". It was the GP, the district nurse and us, in that order, really. So we didn't go into a patient unless we were referred by the district nurses. As a courtesy we would always refer to them. But it did mean on a lot of occasions we didn't have to call the doctor out. Generally, the nursing would change once they had gone into a coma, in as much as the house visits would be more frequent;

phone-calls would take place more often with more visits from our nurses. If we knew the end was very near, we would provide continuous care, as far as we possibly could.

Will: As a case-load you're talking about 35 patients a year, that sort of number? So, to get a sense of the burden on you as a service: what proportion of that number of patients would end up having 24-hour nursing care? That's very intensive input.

Jecca: Actually, very few. We had two occasions when the GP, without consulting us, promised the wife that there would be 24-hour care for her husband. But, of course, we were working for 17 doctors, and the GP didn't ring me to find out if we had other patients, and we had. The Trust had to honour the promise so we had to hire in a private nurse, which was extremely expensive. So, we shared the care. But although I had, on average, around 35 patients a year, it doesn't really mean anything, because with some patients it might have been almost round the clock for three weeks. With another patient, it might have been very much less – just phone calls. That's still a patient, that's still a statistic.

Or, with a dying patient, we might be going in once a day, and the family were coping and wanted to cope, and didn't want us working nights because the son or daughter was there. We had a lot of patients with amazingly caring relatives. And it isn't a criticism of the families who couldn't care, because, of course, some people just can't look after the sick. But I was regularly impressed. The care given by these young members of the family absolutely amazed us, and a lot of them had never cared for a sick person before. There is such a lot of very intimate care you must give at the end. They just wanted to do it. So, we were just in the background then. Often, we would have a young grown up relative sleeping with the parent who was dying, and we would just be downstairs. That happened very often.

Will: There's an interesting set of assumptions there about the idea that, in modern life, somehow there is less expectation that families remain very 'hands on' involved in the end of life care of relatives. Yes, in many ways it is impressive for a family to rally round and care for someone in that setting. But we talked about this at the hospice recently. A new baby requires a lot of care, and in that situation the assumption, very clearly, is that the family must cope. No-one is necessarily deserving of state help for that situation – it's fully expected of you. Yet with a dying patient, it's a different picture. That burden of expectation has been completely taken away. There are all sorts of interesting historical reasons for that, perhaps.

Just going back to some very specific things about that issue of practical nursing needs – this is partly about my ignorance of home nursing. Let's say you have a patient big in size and consequently hard to manhandle. Then add in certain symptoms, let's say you have someone with profuse diarrhoea who is bed bound. How to deal with that situation? Would you take in a hoist?

Jecca: Nurses officially are not allowed to lift any more. So, we had to use lifting devices if they were already in the house. I can count maybe not more than on one hand, patients for whom we had a hoist simply because of the weight of the patient. But in fact, when someone was dying, I personally hated using a hoist. Usually, a second person was all that was needed to move someone heavier.

Will: Usually a relative?

Jecca: Usually a relative, or often I would ring a district nurse and say that, if you are coming, could you come now, and then we would share the task. And if I really couldn't cope, then I would get another one of my nurses. But it's amazing how, at night, when you are on your own, you just do cope. Certainly, I remember a patient who was immensely tall, and it was almost impossible to keep him up the bed. His legs would hang out of the bed, but I put a piece of furniture against his legs at the end of the bed to stop him slipping down. If you were on your own at night, it was very difficult. We had had slide sheets for some time, which are just two pieces of nylon on top of each other. You put one under the patient, and one has got a handle and you pull the patient up. But, of course, the patient slipped down again. The new ones are called something like 'lift and lock'. One side is almost like a Velcro finish. So, you pull them up and in goes the second sheet – it's brilliant. I put it to the test with a man, and his wife and I managed to get these sheets under him. Then, on my own, I lifted him with the handles. Only a couple of inches at a time, but he was so tall, he was a very big weight. And I could do it on my own. It would have been more difficult if I hadn't been as tall, but it was possible. Somehow, putting someone in a hoist when they are dying, is not a comfortable thing. So, we usually got around it with the slide sheets.

Will: Another thing that comes to mind is things coming to a head when someone is in acute distress, perhaps almost at the point of death. In the hospice, the plan involves using a so-called 'crisis pack'. The team will agree in advance essentially high doses of sedating medicines. It was only actually used very rarely, and clearly it is a very different prospect in a hospital compared to being at home. I am wondering if that happened, and how you planned for eventualities like that.

Jecca: You can't say that this is true with every patient, but quite often there was a pattern when someone was dying. I had one patient who, by nature would become quite distressed quite easily. With him I got into a pattern of quite regularly having to give a sedative even while he was on a syringe driver. In many cases you were prepared for the distress at the end. You also get patients who don't show much distress, but can do so at the very end, which is immensely upsetting for the families. I had one patient at night, I remember, when we had to wait a long time for a doctor because he had been called out, and it was very distressing for me, and the patient and her husband. But overall, we could get drugs very easily, and with some doctors, they allowed you to have extra in the syringe driver bag. And if I was to ring a doctor and it was in the middle of a surgery, he would say, "Yes, give it, and I will come by after surgery and write it up." So, it was very rare that we did not have the opportunity to use our discretion as to giving them sedatives. Because, if it really is at the end, it is agonizing for the families: that their loved ones' pain is the image they will be left with.

Will: What happened to that patient?

Jecca: The GP had given her a large dose of morphine, and then had left 2 more specific drugs for me to give if needed. It took most of the night to get her peaceful, and she died the next day.

I had never had a patient who needed that amount of medication to keep them peaceful. That was an incident that upset me greatly, and we had quite a lot of discussion about it afterwards with the GP and the district nurses, because we didn't feel we had done our job properly. But the GP certainly was doing all she could, and it wasn't working.

Will: Even with this lady, was there not discussion about having to send her to hospital?

Jecca: Yes, there was. When the GP came (she was there when I arrived at 1am) she and I had a talk outside, and she said she really wanted to send the patient to hospital. But two of the family members were adamantly against this. She had come home from hospital and had been very unhappy there and had begged her not to let her go back. She was only semi-conscious, and in the end the collective decision was to keep her at home. I think it was the right thing. But it was a very difficult decision. I know the GP did everything she possibly could – for her too it was a very distressing case. But luckily, that didn't happen very often.

Will: Why did you think you hadn't done your job properly?

Jecca: I think because a big part of our job was keeping the distress level for the families to a minimum by keeping the patient peaceful and well nursed and comfortable. Therefore, they could sit quietly with their loved ones and not become distraught by anything they saw. This was a distressing scenario. It's a case that hung quite heavily with me. I suppose we couldn't have done more than we did, but it wasn't a satisfactory conclusion. The family didn't blame us. They didn't blame the GP. They just felt deeply sad that their relative had to suffer in that way.

Will: Do you think there would have been difficulties with that case wherever she was – even if she was in a hospice with other staff on hand? Is it the case that some people are distressed at their death and you can't do anything about it?

Jecca: As a nurse, not having the knowledge of a doctor, I don't see that the scenario would have been any different in a hospice. You may have had more doctors' opinions, but it was the middle of the night so there may not have been many around. I didn't feel worried about that. I suppose, in a way, I would have liked her to go to hospital because it was almost beyond our control. But she didn't go, and so I think, looking back on it, we did the very best we could, but it wasn't great. However, I don't see that it would necessarily have been different in a hospice.

***

Will: A change in tack.

The book, *A Fortunate Man; The Story of a Country Doctor* by John Berger discusses the intimacy of the relationship between doctor and patient, and he says: *"In illness we ideally imagine the doctor as an elder brother or sister. Something similar happens at death. The doctor is familiar of death. When we call for a doctor, we are asking him to cure us, and to relieve our suffering. But, if he cannot cure us, we are also asking him to witness our dying. The value of the witness is that he has seen so many others die (this rather than the prayers and last rites was also the real value which the Priest once had.) He is the living intermediary between us and the dead. He belongs to us, and he has belonged to them. And the hard but real comfort which they offer through him is still that of fraternity."*

What I want to think about here is a different part of looking after someone who is dying. Berger talks about the role of the doctor or the nurse as being a witness – being someone who has witnessed other deaths, and so brings a gravity and authority to the situation as a result. An authority that in other times may have been given to a priest or minister. In terms of thinking back over the time when the home nursing was going, is this role of witness one you identify with? Could you talk a bit about the role over and above purely that of being the nurse?

Jecca: I can identify with that very well, because quite soon after we started, I was very much aware that, when I went in for my first visit to the families, how very quickly they became dependent on you. In the beginning one wondered whether it was because of you as a person, but very quickly I realised it was because, in their eyes, at this very difficult time, they felt the two people who did know what was going on (or what might possibly happen) were the doctor and the nurse. So, they immediately put their trust in you. They probably feel that you know more than you do, but it gives them that confidence to continue their journey with less fear, less apprehension, because you are there to field the difficult times. So, I think the role of nurse is immensely important to the patient, but almost more so for the families.

Will: The phrase you used was 'taking a big responsibility into the house' when you start a case – of being the ones that are going to be relied on. Can you give an example of a case where maybe the nursing needs were very simple, but the sense of reliance, this more abstract role, was very crucial and somehow more testing?

Jecca: I can think of one case where it was a younger person who was dying. The husband wanted her nursed in the sitting room so that if there were ever any visitors or nurses we could all be in the same room together. The nursing was minimal because the patient was by then unconscious. The needs of the family were enormous. I suppose 95% of the time we spent in that house was caring for them, talking to them, being reassuring, giving them the care they needed. Although our primary reason for going in was because somebody was dying, a very large part of our work was the care of the extended family.

Will: You as a nurse have witnessed many people die. Do you think that is significant in this setting, does it carry weight? It is this idea that Berger talks about of the health care worker as bearing witness, a role that he ascribes to a priest in earlier times.

Jecca: I think that is true, because in earlier days the priest would always be present. It's interesting to me that so few people ask to see a priest. But I think it's much more than our just being a nurse in there. For the families it means a great deal that, for us, to witness a death is quite a usual thing, although every occasion is completely different. I have seen it with the district nurses. Some of the district nurses have not always witnessed death, or only rarely if they have. The fact that we are witnessing it all the time adds to the confidence they place in us and gives us the confidence to be there.

Will: So, you are relying on other professionals giving you that role as well as family members giving you that role?

Jecca: Yes. I think I am referring to other professionals as well. In my experience quite a lot of the GPs did not have extensive experience of death, in so far as before we started a lot of their terminally ill patients went to hospital or to a hospice. A tremendous amount of learning took place within the general practices, and in a sense, we grew through it together. Certainly, the district nurses who worked for us felt it had been a very valuable period for them, as they had very much more experience of death in the home through our presence.

As time went on I think the GPs grew in confidence and were much more often in the home, whereas in the beginning we did feel we had been handed the patient, and it was our job to see them through to death. Obviously, they were always involved when it came to prescribing drugs.

Will: Was there a sense in which you felt more experienced than the doctors you were working with?

Jecca: No, I didn't have that feeling right at the beginning, though I had had experience of terminal care with my parents and relatives. At the beginning we were very much learning together, the district nurses, GPs and ourselves. I did arrange for my nurses to have extensive palliative education, monthly meetings with speakers – and after some time I noticed we were calling on the

GPs and the district nurses less and less as we felt increasingly capable of dealing with situations as they arose. There were times, of course, when they both had to become involved. But there were many occasions when we were able to see through a procedure on our own, because that was all we were doing. They were busy with their other patients too, so, for them, their palliative patients were a very small percentage of their workload, whereas for us, that was all we were doing.

Will: In different ways, historically that relationship between doctors and nurses has been quite a complicated one. An example in my experience is of experienced sisters in a hospital setting, junior doctors coming in, and there being this slightly uneasy power relationship between the two. I am wondering if, in the community, this became problematic at all, among different professional groups and everyone wanting to retain control?

Jecca: Yes, to some extent when we started. I think I assumed that the GPs would welcome this new idea of having our team going in at the end of somebody's life. On average we worked for about 16 or 17 GPs, and I noticed quite early on how for some of them our presence wasn't entirely straight forward. It was as if we were taking over, we were taking control of that patient – which of course we never did because we couldn't prescribe, and we were always led in the nursing care by the district nurses. So, in a sense we were always number three down the list. But it took several years for some of the GPs to make us feel they really valued us as part of their team. But that was quite an interesting exercise. Certainly, by the end, we didn't have any problems like that.

Will: You say you were 'number three' in the chain. And yet you and your nurses were those closest to what the actual day to day problems were; you were the front line. Others in that chain of decision making were not so present – can you say a bit about that?

Jecca: I think it might have been more difficult than it actually was, because when we started we had a clear plan of action, and that was that the patient would be referred to us from the district nurse, who had had consultation with the GP. The drugs were all prescribed by the GP, and all the care plans were set up by the district nurses. Right until my retirement that is how we worked, and because it worked so well, we continued in that pattern. But the GPs and the district nurses became more open to suggestions from us about treatment and the changing of drugs. That was how we grew over the years. By the end I really felt the GPs were listening to us. They didn't necessarily always do what we said, but they were keen to have our input. But at the beginning it wasn't so.

Will: Related to this, I am just thinking about some issues to do with how people relate to their work. This is from my experience now. Comparing general medical care and palliative care – there are lots of things that are broadly the same, and then certain things that are very different. One of the things I have found in the hospice is that, over and above the normal engagement that people have with their work, there is something like a feeling of vocation about it. (I can't think of a better word than vocation). When you are looking after the dying there is an element of mission to it. I think this works both ways. There's a good side and a more questionable side. The good side is that it does make people feel very motivated, and I suggest that most of the work done in the field is very good. People are really trying to do their best for this very vulnerable group. I think the flip side of it, though, is that if people have a sort of 'mission' about what they are doing, it can create problems between professional groups, it can create problems between staff members.

I don't know if there are generalisations about this, in as much as, if you are doing something with a mission, everyone is trying to do it 100% right, and also people have slightly different ideas about how it should be done. There are potential areas of friction in that. There are potential areas of friction in every working life, but there is something specific about palliative care where everyone is doing it with a greater intensity maybe. If people fall out, they can really fall out. I don't know if this is something you relate to at all.

Jecca: Comparing hospice work with what I have been doing is very different, because we are in the patient's home. Therefore, in a sense, we are working on our own. We may be in very close touch with the GP and in very close touch with the district nurse. But most of the hours we do in somebody's home we are the only professional there. So, I think falling out with people, is less likely to happen.

We always took enormous care when it came to interviewing the nurses, and of course we had to have CVs and references. But we weren't really all that interested in the CVs because some of the people that came to see us who were extremely well qualified were just not right for this sort of work. And, again, like the work itself, you got better at judging people. I think there definitely is a sense of mission in this work. But doing it in a home, as time went on, the district nurses and the GPs were just relieved to have us there. We made their workloads easier too. We developed a very good team liaison and, really, the minimum friction. But I think that has a lot to do with the fact that it was in the home rather than in a hospital or hospice set-up.

Will: I can see that. It's a very different working environment. But do you think your colleagues in Campden Home Nursing had a sense of vocation? Was it a job of work – an important job of work – but simply a job of work?

Jecca: I think amongst the nursing team, although we were very different people – different ages and stages of life – there was a tremendously strong thread which ran through the whole team whereby we aimed to give the very, very best care to every family we went into. But what helped me tremendously was the support from the Board of Trustees, only two of whom were medical. They all had a burning desire to provide an excellent service, and that, for the nursing team, was a tremendous strength.

Will: Going back to something we were talking about earlier, you made this point specifically, very rarely was the priest or religious person called in. In some ways this is quite a personal thing. I know you have a devout faith; how much of the work was connected to a Christian context for you, what part did faith have to play?

Jecca: That isn't how I 'wear' my faith in a sense. But I truly believe that if I hadn't had the faith I have I wouldn't have been able to do the job I did. There were times when it was very difficult, and I had to hand it over to God. I am somebody who has always found it hard to pray in church because there are too many distractions. I used to pray a lot in my patients' houses, especially at night when it was quiet, privately, to myself, and I feel quite sure I couldn't have done this work without having that strength.

Will: If the family had asked you to pray with them, or if a patient had asked you to pray with them, did you feel like that was just separate to your nursing role?

Jecca: No, I didn't find it particularly separate because it was all so much tied in together for me. I had a patient once, who had just come to live in our area. Within three weeks of his arrival, he discovered he had a large tumour. Within six weeks he was terminally ill. His wife happened to mention that they didn't go to church. I had previously said, as I always did to my families, "If you do want to see a priest you have only got to ask one of the nurses." A few days before he died, his wife asked to see the vicar. He came, and although I hadn't had enough time to tell the vicar anything about this family, he just sat down with this man and talked to him softly about his life and the things he loved doing, about his family and grandchildren. After ten minutes of this, he said, "Would you mind if I said a prayer, to myself, for you?" The couple agreed and asked that he spoke it aloud, which he did. When he left, they both said how pleased they were that he had been.

Three days later when I was back with them, the husband was unconscious. His wife asked for the vicar again. So he came. And, again, the request came to say prayers out loud. The wife saw the vicar to the door, and at that moment our patient died. We had a wonderful service, a real thanksgiving for a life, the wife has been coming to our church ever since.

Will: I suppose I am interested to think more about how it helps you. I mean, obviously it's a very personal thing: you have a faith and it's important to you. I am guessing you have met all sorts of people in the field who are not particularly religious, who are atheists or of different faiths.

Jecca: In difficult situations I pray for strength for myself, to be strong for the family, and I am praying for peace for the patient, understanding for the family, and just really praying that I can be guided in the right direction to be of help at such a difficult time. I really feel that the fact that I had a faith was helpful even if the family I was looking after didn't. And that is why I say I don't think I could have done that job as I did it without the faith I had, because that is what really gave me the strength, on top of the learning and the experience and the education. But I think at the base of it all I just felt strengthened by my faith to go on doing the work. There were times when it was extremely difficult, and I can think of two instances when I felt perhaps, I might have to give it up. But, again, through the strength I received I was able to carry on. Several of my nurses who are also Christians have said the same thing.

Will: What was it that made you consider giving up?

Jecca: It happened during a very busy period; I felt like the nursing was taking over my life. I had just had an accident and broken my leg, and had some time to think. I was running the Trust from home on the telephone and realised I could no longer go on doing the job on my own. And that is when I started to share the job, and that is how it continued until I retired. It was a very good working pattern for both of us.

Will: Remind me – you started in 1990 and retired in 2004. And when was it you started sharing the job with Arlette?

Jecca: I did it for six years on my own, which meant being on call 24 hours a day, 7 days a week, with a month off a year. After the accident I decided it would be better to share the job. We tried doing two weeks on and two weeks off, but that was too tight. We tried doing two months on and two months off, and that was too long. We decided on a month, and that proved to be very satisfactory.

Will: So, for those six years you were basically on call all the time. That does sound, in hindsight, an incredibly onerous situation.

Jecca: I think when I started the Trust, I didn't really know what it was going to involve at all. I'm not a businessperson, I'm not a manager as such. I just had this idea that it would be wonderful to look after people at home who were dying. And, of course, at the beginning we had no nurses, so we had to recruit all our nurses. I don't think it really entered my head to get a deputy at that stage, and the Trust took off much quicker than I thought it would. So, once we got our team of nurses, I ran it, and I went on running it. Perhaps I needed someone else to say to me, "How about you hire a deputy so that you could share the job?" So, it was a mistake, and having helped another three Trusts get started, one of the first things I said to them was: "Don't have just one co-ordinator. Start with two." And, looking back, I should have taken my own advice! But you can be wise after the event.

Will: Just for the record, give us some very specific sense of how onerous the on-call was?

Jecca: You could be interrupted in the day, naturally. Certainly, if we accepted a social invitation it was on the proviso that I might be called out. That was fine with our friends. If it was something like a theatre or a concert, then I would have a nurse on call for me. But in the first years I didn't do that very much, because I felt in a sense honour-bound to be there on call, as that was my job.

Over a period of 24 hours I would receive between two and eight calls. The actual number of times I was called out of my bed at night was probably no more than six in fourteen years. But, occasionally I would be called at night for verbal advice, for reassurance. I think the fact that I could be contacted 24 hours a day gave great confidence to my families. There were cases where, in fact, we didn't have any nursing input into a family. They were looked after entirely by their own family because they knew they had us the end of the telephone should something go wrong.

Will: So over and above the actual time involved in being on the phone or occasional call-outs, you had that cumulative background of always being on call. Was that onerous?

Jecca: Yes, one was very aware of that, even if one was out walking or gardening. Whatever you were doing, you had an ear to the telephone. And of course, there were times when you didn't hear the telephone and the message would go on the answering machine, and you would find that it was quite urgent. All these small things, I think, helped me to realise that it was totally impractical to be the only one on call. And I am sure there is no other job in the medical or any other world where somebody is on call day and night, 24 hours a day.

Will: Well, it used to happen in all sorts of places, but now we are in a very different era.

Interestingly, the book I was quoting from earlier, *A Fortunate Man*, is the story of a country doctor who sort of worked in the same way. He had a GP colleague, but as a consequence he did a 'one-in-two': he was on call 50% of the time, 24/7, which was quite the norm.

I have just one or two more questions to do with the religious aspect of it. My question is slightly crude, and it's related to the fact that the demographic of the patients you were seeing in Gloucestershire is relatively consistent, i.e. white, nominally Church of England. The question I am groping for is, what are the issues that might have arisen, given how you have talked about your faith, if you were looking after a Muslim patient, or someone of a very different cultural, religious tradition? Given that you are someone of faith, and that you have looked after many dying people, did you have experience of different cultural expressions of death, and how did your faith interact with that?

Jecca: Because of the sort of place I live, I never came across a wide variety of faiths, but I did have an experience with a couple who were of the Plymouth Brethren.

When we went into this couple's house, it was bare. No television, no radio, almost nothing in the cupboards, no ornaments, no knick-knacks, no pictures, nothing. They were a very nice couple. We looked after the husband, and then he died. Four nurses went to his funeral, which took place in a hall with people sitting on all four sides of a square room, the coffin in the middle. We were there for an hour and a half. In only two minutes of that time did anybody speak, and I found it quite difficult, though I had been to a Quaker meeting before, so I knew a little bit about it. When I went to visit the wife the next day, we talked about the service, and she just said to me, "The reason I am going to be able to carry on is because of the strength I got from that service." And it made me respectful of what somebody else believed. I gave a lot of thought to it at the time. And, to answer your question, although it's hypothetical because I didn't have anybody of Muslim or other faiths, I would like to think it wouldn't have made any difference at all. People who are dying, and who do have a faith are terribly in need of whatever religion they are in. But that is the only other experience I had, apart from Church of England and Roman Catholic.

Will: That sounds a very interesting scene at that funeral, almost completely in silence. With many other Plymouth Brethren?

Jecca: Masses.

Will: It sounds a fascinating experience; one where silence was a key part. Many people coming together, witnessing this event, and yet not a verbal expression of worship.

Jecca: It was very different. In a sense, I got the benefit of it by thinking about it afterwards. Certainly in my own case and in my own church (I think this is typical of the Church of England) we don't have nearly enough silence. Very often before the prayers the priest will say, "Let's have a period of silence before we pray", and that period of silence is over before you have really begun to concentrate on that silence. And now, recently we went to our Quaker church on an exchange Sunday, and we met for an hour, and I should think there was ten minutes of speaking, and I really cherished that silence. The only time I can say I really experience it in our church is on

Good Friday at the Three-Hour Service, when during each half hour we have quite a long period of silence. So, in a way, looking back on it, I can appreciate it more than I did at the time, because it was something new to me.

***

Will: Tell me a bit more about the bereavement work you did, and the 'after-care'.

Jecca: A very big part of the job for me was the care of the families after the death, and that's an area I have been in for many years, and feel very comfortable with. That is something I am continuing to do through our church, via a bereavement group meeting once a month, almost always with a speaker. It gives me enormous satisfaction. In a sense I feel, through that work, I am using a lot of my experiences in general from Campden Home Nursing. It's a new group we have just started. There are just three of us. Two of us have done bereavement care before, the third person is very experienced in people's losses more generally, of losing jobs, losing houses, bereavements other than losing a loved one. In our community the vicar will go at the time of death, possibly before, arrange the funeral, take the funeral, and do a follow-up visit. But then he is unable to go back again because of the size of his job. And after a few weeks one of us rings the family, tells them who we are, and asks them if they would like a visit. Some say, yes, they would welcome a visit, and some decline the offer. We remember the anniversary of the death, and every October we have really a rather lovely service in our church for anybody in our community who has been bereaved. It's a candle-lit service, and it seems to give the families great comfort: partly the service itself, partly being with each other. So that is something that will carry on.

The amount of after-care we gave the families varied according to each family's needs, but I would say that at least 90% of the families did want you to go back, and indeed, we continued to go back until we felt that they were ready for us to withdraw.

There were one or two families who were just unable to move on in their bereavement and were very reliant on our visits. I can think of one patient in particular. We visited the bereaved wife for eight years until the end of her life. She just stood still, and it was very hard for her. They had a lovely life together, and she just couldn't move on.

Will: How often did you visit?

Jecca: For those eight years there were three of us who visited her, because we three had been involved in looking after her husband. I would say we went about four times a year, but quite often I would get telephone calls in between, and we would have a chat. There were other families that we would visit now and again, maybe up to six months. Some families had nobody when their partner/loved one had died; no relatives. We used to visit those families a little more often.

There were many families who had supportive children and large extended families, which was very often a help. But they also knew that we were always on the end of a telephone, and that I think brought them a certain amount of comfort.

Will: A perhaps contentious question – do you generally get a sense that men or women are better able to grieve?

Jecca: I think, generally, women find it easier to talk about their pain, sadness and grief. I think in a lot of cases with men, they just are sad and grieving, but they find it difficult to put it into words. Some are able to, but I would say, perhaps, in a way, women find it easier. But because of that, perhaps men are the ones that need more visits and more caring, because they find it more difficult to express their grief. Some of them would say that they find it easier to talk to us about it, who they weren't deeply emotionally involved with, rather than their own children who are going through their own grief and pain. And that, I think, is very understandable with all bereaved people.

Will: I know that this is a bit simplistic, but the thing you hint at is that, if you are able to put your feelings into words, then somehow your grief moves and resolves itself?

Jecca: I do see it, and I have an example from not very long ago, when I was walking with someone I knew whose sister died suddenly from a rare condition. They were a big family so she had a lot of family support. She was a very strong person herself. Two months after this event we were walking together, and she said to me, "I had no idea how ghastly this could possibly be. It had never crossed my mind." And that made me think a lot. The answer is, none of us know, and I think, working with the bereaved, people fall into traps so easily, thinking that those who grieve fall into the same category. And of course, they don't, because they are all unique; relationships are so different. Each grief/bereavement is unique and must be treated accordingly. So, everybody's needs are very different. I am not saying that you necessarily move on more because you can talk about it, but I think, perhaps, if you are somebody who is able to cry and let your emotions out and share them with other people, perhaps from time to time the pain is lessened.

Will: You once made the point to me that, if someone grieves in a very prolonged way, then it can be very isolating. The support and acceptance of grief by the people around, might perhaps wane as longer periods of time pass.

Jecca: Yes. I also think back to the situation where (this now goes back to the dying process) as somebody is dying, everyone – the patient included – goes through a sort of grief process. I have experienced families where there has been annoyance and anger, really, that they've in a way prepared for the death, but a week later the patient is still alive, and yet hovering on the point of death. I think that causes a tremendous strain on the families and the children especially, and the grandchildren. But it does happen quite often.

It prompts me to say that the circumstances of death may, or may not, affect the grieving process. But it is not necessarily true that "time heals, and grief subsides."

Will: In a way the advantage you had in looking after people in their homes is that there isn't any sense of imposing any sort of structure. You are there providing a service, and in a sense the life of the house carries on.

Jecca: I think a very important thing to say now is that, not only does the life of the household carry on, but one of our jobs was to impress upon the families that they really were the leaders of this whole case. They were the ones who made the decisions. Obviously, the doctors prescribed the drugs, but everything was done with their consent, and the more the families were involved in making those decisions, the easier it seemed to be when death came, because it wasn't as if we were walking in and taking over, and they were pushed to the background. They were always in the foreground. All the nurses felt very much the same, that the families were the most important people, and they were the ones with the final decision.

Will: I'd like to try and start to bring your thoughts to a conclusion. Having spoken about how you took on this work, lets think also about how you let it go. Even though at the time when you gave it up, which was a year and a half ago now (this conversation took place in 2005), you were very clear about it, you have wondered since then about whether you gave up too soon. You've also discussed whether there was another role for you in the field; the possibility of re-engaging with it in some way. Perhaps you would like to say a few things about that?

Jecca: When I did decide to retire it took an enormous amount of time and thought, and I didn't do it in a hurry. I hadn't been very well, my energy levels were low. I felt it was pulling me down for the first time, and on a wonderful walk we had in Scotland in the October before I retired in the April, I was thinking very hard about it and desperately trying to find an answer. I just had a very clear picture in my mind that it was time for me to hand over. By the time we came back from that holiday I put that into motion, and I finally retired the following April 2004, a year ago. In fact I did later occasionally nurse friends when nurses were not available, but that was the moment I retired.

What did take me by surprise after I had retired was how very difficult I found it. It was as big a bereavement as I have ever experienced in my life, and I am still now, a year later, very surprised how difficult I found it. I don't miss now the physical nursing. But I do still miss the families and that initial contact when you first enter someone's home and meet the dying. By that point, friends have probably stopped visiting, and it's just family, and in some cases just the spouse. They are frightened, and they are lonely, and you suddenly have a big role to fulfil for that family. That is what I miss.

Will: Is it having something concrete, and substantial, to get your teeth into and engage with? Is it a sense of being needed in that way? What is the thing that you miss?

Jecca: I don't know that it's completely clear to me yet. In some ways I just feel I still have it in me to give to those families and to make a difference to them. I don't really feel I made the wrong decision to retire, but it's still very much in the front of my mind. I'm very, very thankful that I did it. It was a very fulfilling period of my life. Perhaps in a way it's the feeling of being needed. But one of the strongest things I felt when I retired was that I suddenly had no identity. I couldn't see what my role in life was any more. It had been such a huge part of my life. Now my life is quite full of other things, things that I enjoy doing. But there's always that part of my heart and mind that is still very much within the Trust, and in a sense would expect it to go on being, as it was such an enormous part of my life.

But watching Campden Home Nursing continue in a very strong and positive way makes an enormous difference. I think it will always be very close to my heart.

This is the end of the transcript of the interview we did in 2005. Jecca wrote the rest of the account below in 2020, as conclusions.

Conclusion

written in 2020

During my first year of running Campden Home Nursing, I came across people who asked me how and why I was happy to look after the terminally ill – the dying. I hope by reading so far, you will understand why, with much help and encouragement, I set up Campden Home Nursing. Having nursed both my parents, I decided that palliative care was what I wanted to do after David left the Air Force and we had settled in Gloucestershire. It seemed to me that there was a need for this type of care that I was able to fulfil as a contribution in line with my vocation as a nurse. I envisaged nursing patients dying from any cause, not just cancer.

Before we moved to Gloucestershire, I had been thinking about the sort of arrangement that might work. I realised that the management was going to be in a community setting centred in Chipping Campden. Here was a marvellous place to start such an organisation. I got the support from the community and we were able to set up a Board of good trustees, including a secretary and treasurer. This enabled me to concentrate on recruiting nurses and organising the team.

In my first year, I raised my cash target of £3,000 and this enabled me to start. Our area of operation – a radius of 7 miles around Chipping Campden – and my estimation of 13 nurses fortunately turned out to be right. Tribute should be paid to the quality of the nurses and their commitment. Some had other jobs but made time to support the team.

Getting to know GP surgeries with patients in our area was an important part of my job. The combination of GP, district nurses and Campden Home Nursing nurses was fundamental in almost all cases. Formal decisions were made by the GP, district nurses and Campden Home Nursing nurses, in that order. However, towards the end of each case, we were there all the time, and therefore witnessed most deaths without additional medical help.

Knowledge of, and experience in, palliative care was becoming more widely spread and we obviously benefited from this. I held monthly meetings with my nurses in my home, which often included talks by palliative care specialists. This enabled the nurses to get to know each other and share experiences, but individual cases were only discussed between me and the nurses involved.

The discipline of not taking work home, or of temporarily closing one case, before going on to another, was fundamental in running Campden Home Nursing. This was advice I received from the outstanding Director of the Edinburgh Hospice, where I volunteered. It stood me in good stead – particularly when I sometimes had five patients to visit in one day.

Many think that if you go into a hospice, you are going to die. However, in my experience, hospices are more than that. They can provide relief for families and comfort before the end of life. Some patients are then happy to leave the hospice and die at home with nursing care. There are advantages if the hospice has its own home nursing team, because it improves contact between nursing home and the hospice. Further, home nursing can free up beds in hospices.

It is often difficult to judge when a terminally ill person is going to die. This can bring problems, for example, when a patient is in hospital or a hospice and the family would like that person to come home or to go from hospital to hospice. My son, Will, working in St Joseph's Hospice and I, experienced the challenge of forecasting time of death. A related problem was to judge when a person was likely to die within a month, which was the criteria for starting a home nursing case in the early days when numbers of nurses were limited. As time went on, we increased the number of nurses, which enabled us to be more flexible.

My faith is essential to me and was truly helpful in running Campden Home Nursing. But rarely, in the 380 cases in my time, was a Minister of Religion involved at time of death. After death however, many patients were honoured in a Christian religious service. Most people in the Chipping Campden area were brought up with a Christian background, but Campden Home Nursing nursed, or would have nursed, a person of any faith or none.

Retiring from Campden Home Nursing was painful, but I saw there was a need for bereavement care. With support from our church, I organised monthly meetings, first in the parish's Little Glebe Cottage and then at my home. The group grew to include 14 people who felt they needed help and I am glad to say that this has now been continued by Campden Home Nursing.

I feel so fortunate that I was able to start Campden Home Nursing as I knew I wanted to continue my nursing and I was in the right place at the right time, with enough energy to tackle care of the terminally ill. It has been a real privilege to run the first of four home nursing teams in our area, and I am so grateful to Arlette Gaskell for joining me as a co-ordinator – the nursing team and I learnt a lot from her wisdom.

I have enjoyed writing this story. Campden Home Nursing will always be in my heart, and it is a special pleasure to see it thriving so successfully. I am truly grateful to be kept in touch with its outstanding progress.

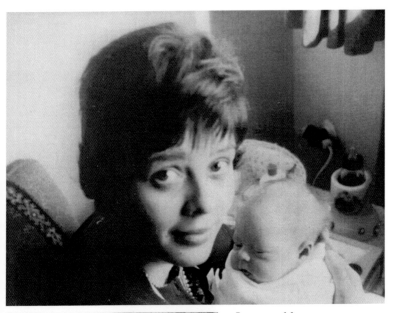

Jecca and her
daughter Julie, 1961

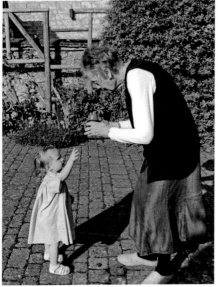

Jecca and little friend,
Bruna

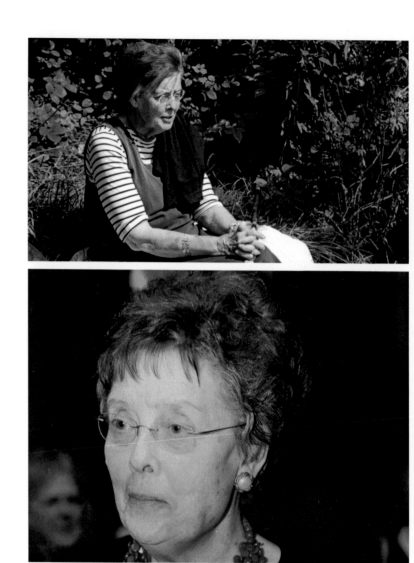

Jecca, 2015 and 2009

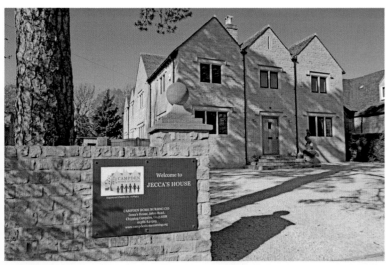

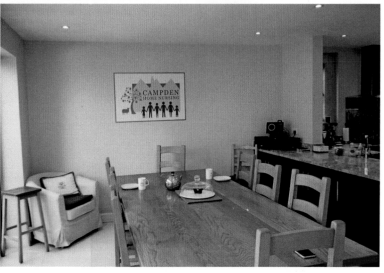

Jecca's House, home to Campden Home Nursing from 2021

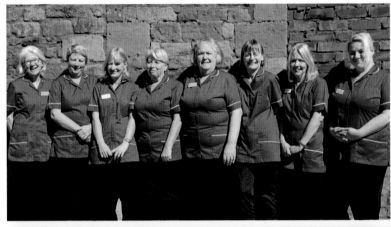

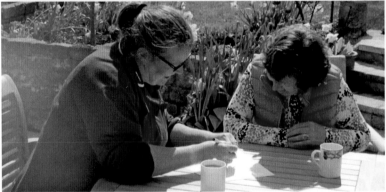

Campden Home Nursing team in action

Memories of Jecca Brook

Helen Makaritis,
CEO, Campden Home Nursing

For those of you that had the joy of knowing her, you will understand what a loss her death is to her family, friends, the charity and Chipping Campden. For those who never had the honour of meeting her, she was the most wonderful, generous lady you could wish to meet with an incredible sense of humour. She started the charity 30 years ago to nurse the terminally ill so they could remain in their own home at the end of life. She would often tell me that she had two great loves in her life, her family and Campden Home Nursing.

All of us in the charity miss her dreadfully. She loved to hear what was happening and of all the developments within the charity, I know that she was incredibly happy and proud of the work our amazing nursing and bereavement teams have been doing and how much the charity has grown to support so many more patients and families over the years. Jecca also loved the shop! She had always wanted a charity shop and was thrilled when we opened it. She visited often and rarely left without buying something!

We will continue to build and strengthen what we have and develop new services in her memory and she will always be there with us in spirit and on the wall of our offices in a lovely new portrait that will now have even greater meaning.

Campden Home Nursing Today

Helen Makaritis,
CEO, Campden Home Nursing

Founded in 1990 by Jecca Brook, Campden Home Nursing has spent the last 30 years providing free registered nursing care to those living with a life limiting illness who, at the end of life, wish to be cared for at home, and holistic support for their families and carers. Our core service is providing Hospice at Home qualified nursing care to the community in and around Chipping Campden. Over recent years our area has increased and we now support 12 surgeries in Gloucestershire, Worcestershire and Warwickshire and give nearly 6,000 nursing hours a year to the community.

In November 2020 we moved into a new property that we have named Jecca's House. The building has our offices, the nurse coordinators hub and bereavement counselling rooms but the main reason for buying this house was to open a Cancer Support Centre for the North Cotswolds. After two years of research we established that there was a need to provide a service that would offer support through one-to-one appointments with an allocated Cancer Support Nurse and activity groups to provide psychological support through a patient's uncertain cancer journey. A program of support events and activities is being planned and a drop-in kitchen established where tea, cake, a friendly face and invaluable support will be readily available.

The team at Campden Home Nursing remains committed to continuing to grow the charity and provide the highest quality of nursing care through our experienced and excellent nursing and counselling teams. We intend to carry on building the charity each year, enabling more people to access the care that they may not be able to access elsewhere, looking after patients, families and carers to the very best of our ability on a daily basis.

Final Thoughts

Julie Brook

Late Fragment
And did you get what
you wanted from this life, even so?
I did.
And what did you want?
To call myself beloved, to feel myself
beloved on the earth.

Raymond Carver

My mother, Jecca Brook, died during a time of immense political turmoil as Black Lives Matters took to the streets all around the world, and we were at the epicentre of the global pandemic.

Reflecting on these huge issues I realise how Jecca was quietly radical in her work, the equality of it, wishing a good end of life for every person.

Death is not easy to think about even though it is an integral part of our lives. Combined with her vocational passion for nursing, Jecca understood the sacred nature of death. The passing from life and the journey this asks of us, unlinking ourselves from everything and every person we love and cherish about life.

She understood that with good nursing care and consideration people are able to have a good death tended by and surrounded by the love of their own relatives at home. That this important time brings laughter, intimacy, revelation in balance with sadness and fear.

She believed that every person was entitled to this kind of nursing care without having to pay for it - irrespective of background or personal and financial circumstances. To enable this Jecca was tireless in her fundraising work to ensure that CHN was managed to a very high standard and that all the nursing staff were paid appropriately. Jecca was equally committed to taking care of bereaved relatives as they navigated the bewildering voyage of grief.

She delighted in the communities she brought together as a consequence of all this work. And she has created a remarkable legacy that goes on flourishing and growing in new places as other communities now follow her inspiration.

Through her own death she gracefully taught us about the essence of her work.

We witnessed the compassionate care of the nurses looking after her in her last days. And we experienced the immense privilege in being present with her as she herself took this final monumental journey.

Acknowledgements

Jecca

I owe so much to Arlette Gaskell, and all the nurses I have had the pleasure of working with for so long. Further, special thanks go to the trustees, chairmen, secretaries and treasurers of the charity. It is due to all their support that I was able to run Campden Home Nursing.

I am greatly indebted to our son, Will, who spent many evenings with me recording our conversation. I am also very grateful to my husband, David, who spent hours putting this story together. Warm thanks also to Jenny Dillon who helped me to draft the Introduction and to Maria Graham-Martin who has done sterling work editing and typing up the story. Many thanks go to her and to Helen Makaritis, the current CEO of Campden Home Nursing for all her support.

Acknowledgements

Will

I'm very grateful to Helen Makaritis, Liz Pyment and Dr Richard Juckes for looking at the text and sharing their thoughts. I am also grateful to Arzu Tahsin for help with editing.

I would very much like to thank Andy Doran and his son and daughter Dominic and Fionnghuala; the case at the start relates to the last illness of their mother Josephine. As will be clear this was a very precious memory for Jecca. I include here Andy's account in bringing the story up to date. I take the view that his generous words provide a fitting conclusion to the book:

"We kept in close touch. The two children have grown up and a granddaughter now shares her grandmother's name. Because of the support of the nurses we as a family had time to plan and to enjoy our remaining time together, and as a couple we were able to talk about what

the future may hold after her death; we even happily planned the order of service together for her funeral. As well as the open door Josephine insisted that I must not live alone. It was a great joy therefore to share in a beautiful wedding not a year after her death with the full blessing of her family. One of the nurses became Godmother to our first child together highlighting how close that friendship had become. My happiness is a direct result of these nurses and the care that we as a family were given when it was most needed.

A month or so before Jecca's death I was invited (instructed) to attend for coffee and spent two wonderful hours reminiscing and discussing life and family etc. I didn't realise of course that that would be the last time we would meet but I am so pleased that we did. Though we couldn't attend her funeral it was a very fitting tribute for us to stand with our fellow Campdonians and honour her last journey along the High Street. Your mother's care of me, my wife and my family at such an incredibly difficult time has enabled me to continue my life in a way that no one would have thought possible at the time."